LIFT 'EM BOOBS

How to achieve fuller and firmer breasts naturally

Kelly Hart

Table of contents

THE BREAST

Women's breasts have been a source of fascination for centuries, but what exactly are they and what do they do? Breasts are made up of fatty and glandular tissue, and are located on the front of the chest.

They are made up of thousands of small glands called lobules, which produce milk when a woman is pregnant or breastfeeding. The milk is then fed to a baby through the nipples. Breasts also contain supportive connective tissue and blood vessels. Breasts come in all shapes and sizes, and no two are exactly alike.

Breasts can range from small and flat to large and full. Breast size is determined by a combination of genetics, body weight, and age.

Breasts can change in size and shape over time, especially during puberty, pregnancy, and menopause. Breasts have a number of important functions.

In addition to providing milk for infants, they are an important part of a woman's sexuality. They can provide pleasure during sexual activities, and can also be used to attract potential sexual partners.

Breasts can also be a source of anxiety for many women. They can be too small, too large, or asymmetrical. This can cause low self-esteem and body image issues

It is important for women to learn to accept and appreciate their breasts regardless of their size or shape.

Taking good care of their breasts, including regular self-exams and mammograms, can also help to ensure their health.

Women's breasts are composed of several different types of tissue. The breast is primarily composed of two large lobes of glandular tissue and fat divided by fibrous connective tissue.

Each lobe contains small glands (lobules) that produce milk (lactiferous ducts). The lobules are connected to the nipple, which is the primary pathway of milk production.

Under the skin, the breast also contains fatty tissue and lymph nodes. The suspensory ligaments of the breasts help to support the glands and the fatty tissue.

The nipple and areola are darker than the rest of the breast and are made up of several types of tissue, including skin, fat, and nerves. The nipple contains a small opening (the papilla) from which milk can be expressed.

The areola is the dark area around the nipple, and it is made up of glands that secrete a lubricant used during nursing. The areola also contains small muscles that can cause the nipple to become erect when stimulated.

The breasts are also composed of blood vessels, nerves, and lymphatic vessels. Blood vessels provide oxygen and nutrients to the cells in the breasts, while nerves provide sensation to the breasts.

The lymphatic vessels help to carry metabolic waste products away from the breasts. The breasts also contain connective tissue, which provides support and structure to the overall shape of the breast.

This connective tissue is made up of proteins, especially a type of protein called collagen.

Collagen helps to give the breast its shape and volume. Over time, the amount of collagen in the breasts can decrease, leading to sagging or drooping of the breasts.

WHY DO BREASTS SAG?

A woman's breasts can sag due to several factors. Age is one of the biggest contributing factors, as the skin's elasticity decreases with age, making it less able to support the weight of the breasts. Weight gain and loss, pregnancy, and genetics can also contribute to sagging breasts.

Weight gain causes the skin to stretch, which can lead to sagging. Pregnancy can cause the breasts to stretch and sag due to the increased weight of the breasts during lactation. Genetics can also play a role in how quickly a woman's breasts will sag.

1. Age: As a woman ages, her breasts may become less firm due to the natural breakdown of collagen and elastin.

2. Pregnancy: During pregnancy the breasts may become fuller and heavier. Once the baby is born and the mother stops breastfeeding, the breasts can become saggy.

3. Weight Loss: Rapid weight loss can cause the skin to lose its elasticity, leading to a sagging appearance.

4. Genetics: Some people are naturally predisposed to having saggy breasts due to the structure and shape of their breasts.

5. Smoking: Smoking can damage the collagen and elastin in the skin and can cause the breasts to sag.

6. Poor Posture: Poor posture can cause the breasts to droop and become saggy.

7. Sun Damage: Excessive exposure to the sun can damage the skin and cause it to become less elastic, leading to saggy breasts.

What to wear to make breasts appear Perkier

To achieve a fuller and perkier appearance for your breasts, there are a few tips you can follow when selecting your wardrobe.

First, choose tops that provide support. This includes bras, tank tops, and camisoles. Bras with underwire, molded cups, and straps that are wide and adjustable are great options. Avoid tops with a lot of stretch as this can cause sagging.

Second, opt for tops that lift and separate. V-necks, scoop necks, and wrap tops can provide a nice lift and accentuate your curves.

Third, look for tops with embellishments such as ruffles, pleats, or other details that draw attention upwards. This can help make your breasts look fuller and perkier. Finally, select tops that have a looser fit around the bust. This helps to create a flattering silhouette and will draw attention away from your chest area. By following these tips, you should be able to find clothing that helps to create the appearance of fuller and perkier breasts.

WAYS TO FIX SAGGY BREASTS

Natural breast enhancement exercises

Natural breast enhancement exercises involve a range of techniques designed to increase the size, shape and firmness of the breasts.

Exercises that may be included in natural breast enhancement programs include chest presses, chest flys, shoulder presses and chest squeezes.

Chest presses are exercises that involve pressing weight away from the body with the palms of the hands. During a chest press, the arms should be parallel with the shoulders and the palms should be facing down. As the arms move, the chest muscles should be tightened and the palms should press against the weights. Chest presses can be done with dumbbells, barbells or a cable machine.

Chest flys are similar to chest presses, but the arms should be held out to the sides, with the palms facing up. As the arms move, the chest muscles should be contracted and the palms should press against the weights. Chest flys can be done with dumbbells, barbells or a cable machine.

Shoulder presses involve pressing weight away from the body with the arms held up at shoulder level. As the arms move, the chest muscles should be tightened and the palms should press against the weights.

Shoulder presses can be done with dumbbells, barbells or a cable machine.

Chest squeezes are exercises that involve squeezing the chest muscles together.

To do a chest squeeze, the arms should be held close together in front of the chest and the palms should be facing each other.

As the arms move, the chest muscles should be tightened and the palms should squeeze together. Chest squeezes can be done with dumbbells, barbells or a cable machine.

Natural breast enhancement exercises can improve the size, shape and firmness of the breasts and can be done with minimal equipment. However, it is important to remember to consult with a doctor before starting any exercise program.

Supplements for breasts enhancement

Natural breast enhancement supplements are dietary supplements designed to increase the size, shape, and firmness of breasts. These supplements are composed of various natural ingredients that are believed to help promote the healthy growth of breasts.

The ingredients in natural breast enhancement supplements are typically herbs, vitamins, minerals, and other plant-based compounds. Herbs such as fenugreek, wild yam, saw palmetto, and fennel are commonly used in these supplements due to their purported ability to stimulate the production of breast tissue. Vitamins and minerals such as iron, zinc, and vitamin E are included to promote overall breast health.

Other plant-based compounds such as phytoestrogens and flavonoids are believed to help promote hormonal balance in the body which can lead to healthier, fuller breasts.

These supplements are typically taken as capsules or tablets and are meant to be taken daily. Some are also available in liquid form. While there is no scientific proof that these supplements actually work, many women report feeling positive results after taking them.

As with any supplement, it's important to speak to your doctor before taking natural breast enhancement supplements. It's also important to research the ingredients in the supplement to make sure that they are safe and effective and to avoid the risk of an allergic reaction.

It is important to keep in mind that these supplements are not a substitute for regular exercise and a healthy diet.

Breast massage

Breast massage is a type of massage therapy that is designed to promote healing, improve circulation, and reduce stress in the breasts. It can be used as part of a larger massage therapy session or as a standalone treatment. Breast massage can help to increase flexibility and range of motion in the breasts, improve lymphatic drainage, reduce tension and soreness, and may even help to reduce the risk of developing breast cancer.

When performing a breast massage, the therapist should always use a light touch and should never use any harsh or aggressive techniques.

The therapist should begin by gently massaging the chest area around the breasts in a circular motion. This helps to warm up the muscles and prepare them for the massage.

Next, the therapist should use gentle kneading and circular motions to massage the breasts. This helps to stimulate the lymphatic system and can aid in the removal of toxins from the breasts. The therapist should then use a combination of soft strokes and circular motions to massage the area around the nipples.

This helps to increase blood flow and can help to reduce any tension or soreness in the nipples.

Use a light, circular motion to massage the area just above the breasts. This helps to improve circulation and can help to reduce any pain or swelling in the area.

Breast massage should always be performed with caution and respect for the client's comfort level. The therapist should be aware of any discomfort the client may be feeling and should adjust the massage pressure accordingly. Finally, the therapist should always use proper draping techniques to ensure the client's privacy and comfort.

Breast massage oils

Natural oils are widely used to massage the breasts for firming. Massaging the breasts with natural oils can help improve circulation, reduce sagging, and improve skin elasticity, resulting in firmer, perkier breasts.

Common natural oils used for breast massage include olive oil, coconut oil, almond oil, and jojoba oil. These oils are rich in antioxidants, which can help protect the skin from damage. They can also help moisturize and nourish the skin, which can improve its overall elasticity and tone.

Natural pastes such as mashed avocado, mashed banana, and mashed papaya are also often used to massage the breasts. These pastes are rich in vitamins and minerals that can help strengthen the skin and improve its elasticity.

When massaging the breasts, it is important to use gentle, circular motions. It is also recommended to use a circular motion with your fingertips and not your nails. Massaging the breasts too vigorously can cause bruising and soreness. It is important to note that while natural oils and pastes can help improve breast firmness, they should not be used as a substitute for regular exercise and a healthy diet.

These methods can help, but in order to achieve the best results, it is important to combine them with lifestyle changes.

Breast enhancement pumps

Breast enlargement pumps are devices that can be used to achieve larger breasts through a process called tissue expansion.

This process involves creating a vacuum around the breasts, which causes the tissue to expand, resulting in increased size. The vacuum created by the pump draws in additional blood flow, which helps to stimulate breast growth.

This can also help to firm and tone the breasts, as well as providing additional volume. With regular use, it is possible to achieve a noticeable increase in breast size. Most pumps use suction cups that are placed over the breasts.

These cups are connected to the pump, which is responsible for creating the vacuum. The vacuum can be adjusted to different levels, depending on the desired effect.

In addition to larger breasts, breast enlargement pumps can also be used to reduce the size of breasts. This is done by reversing the process, creating a vacuum that pulls the breasts back in and reduces their size. Using a breast enlargement pump has a few advantages over other methods of enlargement.

It is a non-invasive procedure that does not require surgery or the use of drugs. It is also relatively cheap, and the results can be seen within a few weeks.

However, there are also some drawbacks to using a breast enlargement pump. There is the risk of developing tissue damage, and the effects are not permanent.

As with any medical procedure, it is important to talk to a doctor before beginning any type of breast enlargement regimen.

NUTRITION AND BREASTS

Breast size is determined by a combination of factors, including genetics, body weight, and hormonal changes. While there is no way to guarantee a specific cup size, a healthy diet and regular exercise can help contribute to fuller breasts.

Nutrition plays an important role in breast health and development. Eating a balanced diet rich in essential vitamins and minerals can help support breast health and enhance breast size.

Consuming a variety of lean proteins, healthy fats, and whole grains can help provide the body with the necessary nutrients to support breast health and growth. Incorporating foods that contain phytoestrogens can also help promote fuller breasts.

Examples of phytoestrogen-rich foods include soy and soy products, flaxseeds, tofu, sesame seeds, and legumes.

In addition to healthy eating, regular exercise is important for overall breast health. Exercise can help tone and strengthen the chest muscles, which can give the appearance of fuller breasts.

Cardio, strength training, and yoga are all beneficial exercises for breast health. It is important to remember that no specific foods or exercises can guarantee a certain cup size.

Eating a balanced diet and exercising regularly can help promote overall breast health, but it is not a guarantee of a certain size.

SMOOTHIES FOR GENERAL SKIN FIRMING

Smooth skin is just as important if you are trying to make your boobs firm and full, because who would want a dull skin and plumpy breasts?

Below are simple smoothies recipes that have been found to be helpful in firming and smoothening the skin.

Tropical Glow Smoothie:

Blend 1/2 cup of frozen pineapple chunks, 1/2 cup of plain Greek yogurt, 1/2 banana, 1 tablespoon of honey, and 2 tablespoons of chia seeds.

Tropical Glow Smoothie is an excellent source of vitamins and minerals that can benefit the skin in many ways. It contains antioxidants that help protect the skin from environmental toxins and free radicals. It is also rich in vitamins A, C, and E, which can help to boost collagen production, improving skin elasticity and firmness. This smoothie is high in fiber, which helps to keep your digestive system healthy and running smoothly, further promoting healthy skin.

All of these vitamins and minerals also help to reduce inflammation, which is a major factor in skin aging. Finally, the smoothie also contains healthy fats that help to nourish the skin from the inside out, keeping it looking and feeling youthful.

Avocado and Cucumber Smoothie:

Blend 1/2 avocado, 1/2 cucumber, 1/2 cup almond milk, 1/2 cup spinach, 1/2 banana, and a handful of ice cubes.

Avocado and cucumber smoothies offer a number of benefits for firming the skin. Avocado is a rich source of healthy fats and antioxidants, which can help to reduce the appearance of wrinkles and fine lines. It's also packed with vitamins C, E, and K, which are essential for healthy skin.

Cucumbers are also high in antioxidants and a good source of silica, which can help to improve skin elasticity, reduce puffiness, and make the skin look firmer and more toned. By combining the two, you get a nutrient-rich drink that can help to improve your skin's appearance. The hydrating benefits of the cucumber can help to lock in moisture, keeping your skin soft and supple. The combination of these two ingredients in a smoothie can help to provide your skin with an all-natural, nutrient-rich boost.

Papaya and Aloe Vera Smoothie:

Blend 1/2 cup of papaya, 1/2 cup of almond milk, 1 tablespoon of aloe vera gel, 1 tablespoon of honey, and a handful of ice cubes.

A papaya and aloe vera smoothie is an excellent way to firm and tone the skin. The combination of these two natural ingredients provides a powerful combination of vitamins and minerals which help to promote healthy, glowing skin.

The papaya is high in vitamin A, which helps to reduce wrinkles and fine lines, while the aloe vera is packed with antioxidants that help to protect the skin from environmental damage. The smoothie is also rich in essential fatty acids, which help to keep the skin hydrated and smooth. The smoothie also contains enzymes that help to break down dead skin cells, which helps to improve the overall texture of the skin. Finally, the smoothie contains anti-inflammatory properties that help to soothe and reduce redness. All in all, a papaya and aloe vera smoothie is an excellent way to promote healthy and firm skin.

Blueberry and Coconut Smoothie:

Blend 1/2 cup of blueberries, 1/2 cup of coconut milk, 1 tablespoon of honey, 1 tablespoon of flaxseed powder, and a handful of ice cubes.

Blueberry and coconut smoothie is a great way to firm the skin. Blueberries are rich in antioxidants which help protect the skin from free radicals and the aging process. They also help increase collagen production, which helps keep skin looking firm and youthful.

Coconut is also packed with healthy fatty acids that help to lock in moisture and keep skin hydrated. The healthy fats in coconut can help to reduce inflammation and soothe irritated skin. Together, blueberries and coconut provide essential nourishment to the skin, leaving it feeling firm and healthy.

Kale and Kiwi Smoothie:

Blend 1/2 cup of kale, 1/2 kiwi, 1/2 cup of almond milk, 1 tablespoon of honey, and a handful of ice cubes.

Kale and kiwi smoothie is a great way to firm the skin and help it look its best. This superfood smoothie is packed with vitamins, minerals, antioxidants, and anti-inflammatory agents, making it a powerful way to nourish and protect your skin.

The antioxidants in kale and kiwi help to fight free radicals, which can cause wrinkles and other signs of aging.

The vitamins and minerals found in these two ingredients help to boost collagen production, which is important for maintaining skin firmness. The anti-inflammatory properties of both ingredients help to reduce inflammation, which can also contribute to aging skin.

Finally, the high water content in kale and kiwi helps to hydrate and nourish the skin, leaving it looking and feeling softer and more supple.

Acai and Pomegranate Smoothie:

Blend 1/2 cup of acai berries, 1/2 cup of pomegranate juice, 1 tablespoon of honey, 1 tablespoon of flaxseed powder, and a handful of ice cubes.

A smoothie made of acai and pomegranate is an excellent choice for firming the skin. Acai is a highly nutritious berry that contains powerful antioxidants, which help to protect the skin from sun damage and premature aging.

Pomegranate is rich in vitamin C, which helps to firm and tone the skin. The combination of these two ingredients also helps to reduce inflammation, boost collagen production, and promote healthy skin cell growth. The smoothie is packed with essential minerals, vitamins, and fatty acids that help to keep the skin hydrated and nourished. The natural antioxidants in the smoothie help to protect the skin from free radical damage, and the omega-

3 fatty acids provide deep hydration that helps to

keep the skin firm and healthy.

CONCLUSION

Accepting your breasts the way they are is an important part of self-love and self-care. Having unrealistic expectations of how your breasts should look can lead to feelings of inadequacy and low self-esteem.

It is important to recognize that every woman's body is unique and that there is no right or wrong way for breasts to look.

The importance of accepting your breasts the way they are is rooted in body positivity and self-acceptance. It is important to recognize that each body is a unique shape and size and that no two bodies are the same.

Accepting your breasts the way they are can help to reduce feelings of insecurity, shame, and guilt. When women learn to accept and love their bodies, it can have a positive effect on their overall wellbeing. It can also help to reduce body image issues and the pressure to conform to beauty standards.

Finally, Learning to love and accept our bodies can help to reduce the risk of developing anxiety and depression. breasts size does not really matter when it comes to sex appeal and beauty. Accepting your breasts the way they are can help to create a healthier relationship with your body and foster a sense of self-confidence

45

and self-love.